HOPE During Cancer Treatment

Surviving and Thriving Through Cancer Treatment

By

J Ewing

HOPE During Cancer Treatment

Table of Contents

HOPE During Cancer Treatment

Port

Neulasta®

Sleep/Naps

Germ Prevention

Alternative Therapies

Attitude

Prayer and Meditation

TV/iPad/Kindle/Smart Phone

Social Contact

Exercise

Diary/eMail Updates/Journaling

Gratitude

How Family and Friends Can Help

Local Support Groups

Professional Counseling Support

Other Support Organizations and Resources

Epilogue

Disclaimer

Please consult your physician regarding your care or before following any of these guidelines or suggestions. Everything contained here relates to my personal experience, but should be reviewed with your physician before implementing.

I have no financial relationship with any vendor or provider noted in this book. Please find the best vendor or source for your needs.

I do not claim any cures but reflect only my personal experience. I do not intend to imply that following any or all of my suggestions will guarantee a cure for your cancer.

I do not expect you to agree with anything or everything I say or recommend. Take what you value and leave anything else behind.

I use the ® symbol for any company or entity noted in this book. I acknowledge their brand and legal protection of their rights. I use this universal symbol so as not to misrepresent whether they are legally trademarked or copyrighted.

Forward and Introduction

I was diagnosed with incurable stage IV Non-Hodgkin's Lymphoma. This diagnosis didn't happen automatically or without a lot of suffering in the process. I experienced eighteen months of chronic pneumonia and drastic weight loss (130 lbs. down to 100 lbs.) and digestive problems before they were able to pinpoint and diagnose the underlying cause. It wasn't until they had to remove my entire left lung due to the considerable damage caused by infection that they were able to find the lymphoma.

I have a lot of wisdom to share. I have been hospitalized numerous times, and I have undergone six months of chemotherapy. I am now living to tell that cancer does not have to be a death sentence. I currently have no active cancer in my body.

I want to share my experience, strength, courage and hope with you. I want to share my advice so that you, too, may survive and overcome chemotherapy or other cancer treatments, and hopefully a life without cancer.

When I was first diagnosed with cancer, I had all of the usual reactions. I went into shock. I was told numerous times to "get my affairs in order." My life became a roller coaster ride with huge ups and downs.

I did get my affairs in order. I updated my Will, Living Will Directive and got my affairs in order to prepare for death. Then I walked my mother and kids through my documents to make sure they were protected and knew of my wishes and where my important documents were located. I gave my valuables to those I wanted to have them. I prepared for death as much as possible. I had my cremation ceremony planned and ready.

Before and after my diagnosis I wasn't living life, and certainly not with joy. I was trying to manage a series of horrible circumstances, namely major illness, and initially I was not managing them well. I was drowning in bad situations. I could barely manage day-to-day survival. I didn't want to be here anymore. I wanted to die. How could I want to stay alive when I felt horrible and sick all of the time and I couldn't engage in life or activities? I was confined to my bed when I wasn't working (if and when I could manage that), my finances were in "free fall" and then I had the dreaded cancer diagnosis. It was more than I could bear, and I was lonely and depressed. Sound familiar? Isolation and depression are very real when you are ill or undergoing cancer treatment or other chronic illnesses.

So, when I was told I had cancer, I chose to surrender to life and to healing. I had no physical, emotional or spiritual strength left. I didn't know how I was going to survive or manage treatment. The age old adage "life will never give you more than you can handle" is one of the worst myths in my opinion. I believe it is actually the opposite. Life will give you MORE than you can handle to break down the limitations we have created to living a life of joy and wellness.

My new oncologist was wonderful and amazing. During my first visit, she recapped my medical history for me so that I knew she understood all I had been through. Initially I was diagnosed with stage II lymphoma. They were going to just "wait and watch" without any further treatment. But after multiple tests, they found additional cancer in my stomach and spleen. This moved me to stage IV. At that point she told me chemotherapy was needed to protect and preserve my stomach. Keep in mind this was one month after major surgery to remove my lung. I was weak, feeling intense pain, and weighing in at 100 lbs. She looked at me and said "you CAN do this and handle this, and you WILL."

It was at that moment that I became willing to live through chemotherapy and survive.

I "saddled up" to take on this experience and to come out the other side a healthier and better and happier person. I believe that is why I am here today. I want to share how I managed the process and am alive and well to tell the tale.

The most important part of the process, that I do not tell enough about in this book, but I will in my next, is the importance of *believing* I would survive and heal.

Every day I would thank God (or your higher power) for the experience of true healing. I prayed this over and over again. I looked at my body in wonder and marvel and I thanked it for healing. I sent my body feelings of love and healing, and thoughts of healing energy. I truly believe this is why I am cancer-free today. Then, all of the right people kept showing up to assist me in my healing journey. I love and thank every one of them. I also thank my doctors and the medical community for the new and fantastic chemotherapy that destroyed my cancer cells but left my other cells unaffected, and actually boosted my immune system.

Important Note: I was very fortunate – if there is such a thing – to have been diagnosed with a cancer that is utilizing a very new chemotherapy and immunotherapy regiment that builds up the immune system (instead of destroying it) and targeted only certain protein receptors and cells. So I did not have to experience some of the worst side effects of traditional chemotherapy. I did not lose my hair, I did not experience anemia or mouth sores. However, I have learned many things from friends, family and co-cancer patients that I will share here. Also, it's important for you to know that many of my prior experiences were similar to my cancer diagnosis, and so I incorporate my shared healing experience of being in the CCU twice, near death pneumonia and toxic shock from infection, major thoracic surgery to remove my lung, and then chemotherapy. My suggestions for all are incorporated here.

I believe that living an authentic and healthy life must incorporate a complete mind-body-spirit healing.

Fear kills. Fear of anything or everything causes stress and disharmony in your mind, body and spirit. This is how I came to my mantra of "live fearlessly." This helped me to learn to live in joy and peace knowing without any doubt that everything would always be handled for my highest good. Everything I needed would be provided to me. I came to know I am valuable to this world. I am meant to be here for a purpose. We all are. I quickly learned to love and accept my cancer because I knew fearing it or hating it would only intensify its power over me. Knowing and believing this without any doubt gave me the strength and determination I needed to surrender and allow the process of healing to work for me.

This cancer experience may be your chance to break through the barrier of your mind and the limitations you have placed on life. If you will surrender to healing, you may experience the greatest transformation of your life. You may then begin to experience an authentic life allowing joy and peace to seep in and be your new reality.

I learned a lot along the way about how to cope and manage life during this process. This is what I want to share with you. This is my healing gift to you. It is my hope that any one or all of these things I learned will help you on your healing journey, too.

Out of life's greatest adversities and challenges often come the greatest joys and accomplishments. Imagine the feeling of knowing that if you can overcome cancer, there is nothing you can't overcome.

Go forth and live fearlessly!

Jennifer

Planning

I don't believe there is anything you can plan for when you hear cancer and chemotherapy and/or radiation as a diagnosis. Your mind might race, go into shock, disbelief and everything may then go into slow motion. There are so many things to manage and consider. It can be overwhelming, and yet your initial survival instinct may be either to withdraw in shock or move into action. Both of these reactions are perfectly normal. You may also experience anger, sadness, fear and dread. These, too, are normal feelings.

Throughout the process I was flooded with phone calls and emails from family and friends. They were so heartwarming, but I also became overwhelmed with how I would respond to everyone. There weren't enough hours in the day to call everyone, especially when I didn't feel well and I was very low on energy. Some days the news was so unpleasant or complicated, I didn't want to keep repeating it. I solved this problem by:

Sending email "updates" whenever there was a development;

And/or, creating a Facebook® page where everyone could share, and I could post my updates, too.

Legal and Financial

I encourage you to make sure that your Will, Living Will Directive, and Power of Attorney are updated. If you do not have these, I recommend you create and complete them. The hospital or infusion center will ask for a Living Will Directive. Having these updated will just make everyone more comfortable if everything is in order.

If you do not have these documents created and filed, then you are at the mercy of your state's probate laws. Don't go there. If you don't specify your desires, the state will specify for you. They will declare who gets your assets based on state laws after months or years of proceedings. Please visit an attorney to have this done, or seek a competent online resource like www.legalzoom.com. This is especially important if you have minor aged children. If you have life insurance or retirement assets, please make sure the beneficiary information is complete and up to date.

It is important that you share these documents and your wishes with your primary family members and caregivers. This will reduce their anxiety and will help everyone be prepared and settled.

I also set up my monthly payment obligations via online bill pay through my bank. I set up my payments for six months on the same date so that I didn't have the stress or worry about knowing if my payments were made. If you want another option, use Quicken Bill Pay® to establish regular monthly payments through your bank.

If these options are still a challenge, or not an option, then please have your lawyer prepare a "Power of Attorney" to assign these obligations to a trusted family member or friend. This will also be crucial in the implementation of a life insurance claim, too. (I'm not trying to be pessimistic, but I want you to "cover all of your bases.")

If moving into treatment will put you out of work and onto disability, then first seek your Human Resources department if you have one. They will be able to clearly tell you what benefits you have, and how they work.

If you do not have short or long term disability insurance through work, you may be eligible for Social Security Disability Income. Go to www.ssdisabilityapplication.com to begin the process.

Finally, call your Human Resources Department to understand your leave of absence rules, disability requirements, and make arrangements for your work schedule during treatment.

Create a Plan

Assess your situation. I was single and living alone. I had unique challenges in how to manage my life situation. You may be married, have children, or both.

Consider your resources. Can you create a schedule and map out requests from family, friends and neighbors? If you have children, I would recommend creating a calendar of activities and events. Call parents of children in the same activities to have them carpool for you.

If you are single, map out a calendar of treatments and reach out to friends or family and assign them "dates of service" to help you drive to and from treatments or procedures. If you need overnight care, plan that into your calendar. They are more than willing to help – *you just need to ask.*

If you do not have family members to rely on during this time, check your local community resources. There are public and private organizations that will drive you to appointments or run errands for you as needed.

Fever

If you are undergoing chemotherapy, there is a high probability that your immune system may be suppressed and unable to fight infections. Your oncologist wants to know as soon as an infection develops to prevent toxic shock or other complications involved with an infection.

You will be encouraged to call your physician anytime of the day or night if you develop a fever of 100.5 degrees or higher. If so, call their number and request an immediate call-back. They will instruct you on what to do with a fever.

Try to get in the habit of washing your hands regularly. This will help eliminate germs that you might contract regularly. (*See my chapter on Germ Contamination and Prevention.*)

I encourage you to keep several clean thermometers. (*See my "Travel Survival Kit".*)

Note: Many of my suggestions in this book are designed to reduce your exposure to infections. I cannot predict them all, but the purpose of this book is to help you eliminate your risk as much as possible.

Diet

When undergoing chemotherapy or other treatments, focus on eating and drinking what you can and when you can. I believe it is important to eat as many natural foods as possible, and reduce or eliminate processed foods. You also need to stay hydrated so drink plenty of water or high quality fluids. You also need to disregard some well-meaning family or friends who may act out of concern and pressure you to eat more than you can, especially if you have lost weight. It is important to keep your body functioning at its best possible capacity, but forcing more than you can handle may only cause more complications. As a rule, focus on eating natural foods and minimizing processed foods. This way, the food will be more nutrient dense and easier for your body to digest. Also, ask your physician to guide you about any diet restrictions you may have. (*See my section on High Calorie Supplements.*)

Tip: All hospitals have a nutritionist. I highly encourage you to utilize them. They will provide excellent guidance on how to manage your given situation. I did and they were excellent. Ask your physician to order this for you. It should be covered by your insurance.

Tip: Chemotherapy can impact the center of the brain where hormones and appetite are controlled. My oncologist told me that I may feel very similar to being pregnant for this reason. You may experience strange food cravings and food aversions. This is not a cause for alarm or concern. Adjust your diet accordingly.

Nausea

Nausea is a very common condition from chemotherapy, and also from many symptoms of cancer. It is a grueling condition to deal with, but fortunately, there are solutions.

Rubbing Alcohol: A nurse taught me to carry alcohol swabs. These are the kind they use before an injection or IV. If you feel nausea starting, open the swab and breathe in the alcohol. *(Note: this is rubbing alcohol, not the drink.)* This will usually end light swells of nausea.

Rubbing alcohol on a cotton swab at home works well. Just take a couple of sniffs.

Lemons are incredible for eliminating nausea. Squeeze juice from a half of a lemon and warm in good water. *(See my chapter on Lemons.)*

If you are on the road, and don't have access to anything else, suck on Peppermint Altoids®. Peppermint is very soothing and is said to remove nausea. I learned this from my physical therapist.

Ginger is said to be a good cure for nausea, but I caution you that ginger is very pungent and strong. It can counteract your nausea if you are too liberal with its use. I suggest a small slice of fresh ginger, and a slice of well cleaned lemon in a hot water tea of peppermint or chamomile. Use Stevia if you need any sweetener.

(Note: tradition has said to drink to ginger ale for stomach discomfort. Most commercial ginger ale does not contain natural ginger and contains high fructose sugar and a bunch of toxic chemicals. I do not drink this.)

Make your own ginger ale by adding fresh ginger and lemon steeped in water and added to sparkling water and stevia. Add lemon and frozen grapes for a kick.

Finally, there are very good pharmaceutical anti-nausea medications. Ask your doctor to prescribe one for you to manage serious or chronic nausea.

Food and Menu Choices

Once I knew I was going to undergo chemotherapy, I made it my first priority to make several meals that I could freeze and have ready so that I could have complete healthy meals without further preparation while I was undergoing treatment. I wanted to create meals that were healthy, contained all of my daily calorie and nutrition requirements, and most importantly, would be easy on my stomach and satisfying. I didn't want to come home from treatments feeling exhausted, nauseous or emotionally drained worrying about what I would eat and having to fix it.

I spent a week making these meals, and fortunately I had friends and family to help.

Tip: If you are a friend or family member looking to support and help someone going through chemotherapy, this would be a very good choice for you to help your loved one.

Tip: Ziploc®, Hefty® and many other brands offer 2 or 3 section sealable containers that are freezer and microwave safe. I highly recommend these since you can create an entire meal portion and freeze to save for instant heating and serving. You can find these at your major grocery store, www.amazon.com, or another internet site. I strongly recommend glass containers since they are much safer and healthier for reheating and serving, but you can use the plastic versions for convenience if necessary.

Tip: If you are going into the hospital, I encourage you to have these made ahead of time if possible. Your caregiver can bring a container meal to you to heat at the hospital. This will help you overcome the hospital food problem. I could not eat or welcome the food from the hospital. Knowing I had food I could eat was SUCH a help. Most hospitals have a family station with a microwave. If not, most nurses would be happy to microwave for a patient. (Note: Hospitals may have a policy where only a patient can eat in a patient's room, and caregivers may be asked to go to a waiting or sitting room to eat their food. This is not intended to be isolating, but rather a quality protection.)

You can make your favorite foods and meals by having different compartments. Make your favorite main course. Add a cooked vegetable and a grain like quinoa or boiled red potatoes with vegan butter and parsley, or baked sweet potato. For lunch, prepare a hummus plate with pita and olives/feta/cucumbers, or tuna with crackers and fruit and fresh vegetables. (*Note: These lunch plates cannot be frozen. They need to be fresh, but your caregiver can bring them to you.*)

Tip: For friends or family, please ask what they want and can eat. There may be diet restrictions or food aversions. Don't assume your favorite food or chicken noodle soup.

Recipes

These recipes are easy to make, nutrient dense, filling and easy to prepare and freeze. They are also easy on the stomach. I kept these on hand in individual containers to heat and eat anytime.

Senegalese Chicken and Peanut Soup

This is a high calorie, nutrient and protein dense soup that will serve as a meal. It is easy on the stomach and digestion, and provides satiety. You can expect 1200+ calories from a bowl of this soup.

(Don't let the onions and spices fool you. Contrary to common sense, many spices are actually soothing and helpful for your stomach and digestion. Turmeric is an incredibly healthy spice and is indeed being researched as a potential cancer fighting agent.)

This is really very gentle on the stomach. Often when I could eat nothing else, I ate this soup and it tasted so good. If you have any dietary restrictions, feel free to omit or make modifications. It will still be delicious. This freezes very well, so make a large pot and freeze in individual containers. (I used to serve this in my boutique catering business, too.) This is so easy to make. It is one of my all-time favorite soups.

Note: If you are making this in the spring or summer, skin the sweet potatoes and place in the crock pot to cook with the soup. In the fall and winter, use butternut squash. Buy the already peeled and diced squash. If you are vegetarian, omit the chicken and use vegetable broth. I have found that alternate nut butters do not bring enough flavor or density. Use peanut butter if your diet allows. You can go very heavy on the squash or sweet potatoes but may need to adjust seasonings for flavor and taste.

Ingredients (Serves 8)

1-2 lbs. of diced skinless chicken
1 onion, chopped finely or coursed in a food processor
2 cloves of garlic, minced
1 tsp. cayenne pepper
2 tablespoons of sesame oil
2 tablespoons of curry powder
1-2 teaspoon of turmeric
58 oz. chicken or vegetable stock (or broth)
1 cup water
6-8 cups sweet potato/butternut squash chopped
58 oz. can of petite diced tomatoes
1 ½ cups peanut butter
28 oz. unsweetened coconut milk
Salt and pepper to taste

In a slow cooker, add all ingredients except peanut butter and coconut milk. Cover. Cook on low temperature for 6-8 hours, or 2-3 hours in the oven at a low temperature (300 degrees). Uncover to let rest.

In a bowl, whisk coconut milk and peanut butter. Stir into soup. Simmer for 30 more minutes.

If texture is an issue (as it was for me), then you can blend this in a food processor for the same taste and nutrients.

Best Fast Meal: Miso Soup

I have learned and I am of the mindset that soy products should be avoided, unless they are fermented. If soy products are fermented, they are actually outstanding protein sources, and bypass the problems of negative health effects from soy causing hormones or GMO (genetically modified organism) problems.

I discovered Miso by accident when I had to endure colonoscopies, upper endoscopies and CT scans that required me to fast after midnight but I could drink clear liquids. You know the drill: you're hungry and thirsty, but you can only drink clear liquids, and just knowing you can't eat only makes you "hungrier and thirstier!"

I had a can of white Miso paste in my refrigerator from a recipe I wanted to make. I made a cup of quick Miso soup on a day of a procedure and WOW! It really satisfied me, got me through the procedure, and now I drink it regularly. I especially drink it at night before bed. It's warm, satisfying, and delicious, and it takes away any sense of hunger. It is a good protein source and it is very healthy.

This is also very soothing on the stomach. I took this with me to chemotherapy sessions to drink and satisfy me and to help prevent nausea from coming up.

Buy a jar of white Miso paste. I find it in the refrigerator section of the grocery store where health foods are sold. An always guaranteed option is Whole Foods® or Wegman's®.

Put a tablespoon of Miso paste in a coffee cup with a teaspoon of vegetable or chicken concentrate or bouillon. Add water and microwave for 2 minutes. Mix and enjoy. If you are having a procedure that requires liquids only, place the soup through a strainer to catch the miso pellets. Otherwise, I make a container and keep it in a glass container in my refrigerator to have on hand at all times. It's delicious.

Tip: I bought a few small glass bottles of tea. When I was done drinking the tea, I cleaned the bottles in the dishwasher and used them to make and store miso soup in the refrigerator. They were ready to grab and go.

Fresh Green Soup

This is best in spring and summer

4 tablespoons of butter or olive oil
2 onions coarsely chopped
2 pounds of zucchini coarsely chopped
2 pounds of cucumbers (non-waxed), seeded and
coarsely chopped with skins
3 cups of chicken broth or vegetable broth
¼ cup of fresh dill or 2-3 tablespoons of dried dill
Salt/pepper to taste
1 lemon

Melt butter or oil in a deep pot. Add onions. Cook over medium heat for 10 minutes or until onions are sweating but do not brown. Add broth and vegetables. Cook for 20-30 minutes on low heat until vegetables are soft. Cool to room temperature. Pour into a blender with dill and blend until smooth. Serve warm or chilled. Sprinkle fresh lemon juice when serving. This soup keeps well in the refrigerator or freezer. This soup is a crowd pleaser.

Easy Anytime Chicken Vegetable Soup
(Serves 8)

1 lb. chicken (any part) without skin (with or without bones)

1 bag cabbage and carrot coleslaw
½ zucchini chopped
½ cup fresh or frozen organic corn (optional)
1 clove of garlic minced
2 stalks of celery chopped
28 oz. can of chopped tomatoes
2 tablespoons of fresh parsley (1 tablespoon of dried)
1 teaspoon of dried thyme and basil
1 bay leaf
4 cups of chicken stock
Any other optional vegetables you enjoy (peas, green beans, carrots, lima beans, etc.)
Salt/pepper to taste
Lemon

In a soup pot, put all of the ingredients (except lemon) in the pot, and bring to a boil. Lower heat and simmer for 1 hour. Remove any chicken bones or skin that might have been added. Chop or shred chicken if necessary. Adjust seasonings to taste. Sprinkle with fresh lemon juice when serving. This soup keeps well in the refrigerator or freezer.

Vegan Butter

(Note: Before I went into chemotherapy, I ate a very highly processed food diet. Once I decided to accept healing, I changed my diet drastically to a natural based food diet. Due to the digestive issues and stomach damage, my doctor recommended limiting dairy products. I am so glad I did, because I found that I had a different favorite taste by getting good fats with a lot of flavor. Now that I have regained my natural weight, my body feels full in ways it never did before. I have better muscle mass and my natural fat spots (i.e. breasts, buttocks) are full and firm in ways they never were before cancer. I attribute this to my natural foods and my healthy oils. See below for the vegan butter I now use for just about everything.

This is a delicious and healthy alternative to butter or other fats for vegetables or bread. This is a way to get good quality oils in your diet. Simply mix together and keep in your refrigerator. Use it just like butter or oil.

In a container mix together:

1/3 cup coconut oil

1/3 cup flax seed oil

1/3 cup extra virgin olive oil

2 tablespoons of nutritional yeast

(This can be found in bulk at Whole Foods® or a health food store. This has a buttery flavor and is high in vitamin B12.)

½ teaspoon onion and garlic powder

Salt/Pepper to taste

Smoothies and Juice

Smoothies or fresh juice are an excellent way to add key vital nutrients and satisfy hunger. There are two types of juice: Juice extractors that pull the juice out of fruits and vegetables, or a whole food blender.

(Note: Beware of smoothies in some commercial establishments. They are often just frozen concentrates with a lot of sugar. Ask for the actual ingredients before ordering.)

Tip: I contribute an enormous amount of my healing and regaining energy, strength and ideal body weight to whole food blending and juicing.

Juice (From a Juice Extractor)

You can combine any combination of fruits and vegetables to prepare your juice. Carrots make a great base for juice. You can simply pick the fruits or vegetables you want to add and create your favorite juice.

Do not juice bananas, avocadoes, skins of citrus fruits or fruit pits. Bananas and avocadoes are thick and will junk up your machine. There is not enough juice to extract. Skins of citrus fruits are bitter and do not contain juice, either.

You can also add super green concentrates or super food powders to enhance your juice.

Whole Food Blending

I prefer whole food blending in a high power blender to create smoothies and soups that are fresh, delicious and nutrient dense but easy to digest. (I use a VitaMix® Blender but there are other good blenders on the market, too, like Nutri Bullet® or Blend Tec®.)

There are numerous recipes on the internet, or many books dedicated to creative recipes. Here are a few tips on how I manage my daily food preparation. My goal is to prepare at least one whole food meal for breakfast. I also use this to supplement other meals for soups, too.

Buy 1-3 fruits or vegetables that are in season and keep them in the refrigerator for daily use. Clean and prepare them so they are ready for use.

Keep out of season fruits and vegetables in the freezer to use as additions and enhancers.

Use rice milk, coconut milk or almond milk as the liquid component of drinks or soups. I also use Aloe Vera juice because it helps aid digestion and does not mask the flavors of juice. You can use plain or vanilla yogurt if you are not dairy sensitive.

Add 1-2 tablespoons of ground flax seeds or chia seeds to each drink. (*It is important that flax seeds be ground or they are useless. If your machine will not completely grind the seeds, then use a clean coffee grinder instead.*) Chia seeds do not have to be ground.

Keep fresh grapes in a container in the freezer to use as the "ice cubes" for drinks. They also act as a natural sweetener. Put your bananas in the freezer to keep longer and to chill your drink. I also buy farm fresh tomatoes in the summer and place them in an airtight bag after cleaning. I pull them out as needed to use as fresh tomatoes (note they should be in the refrigerator for a few hours to thaw before they can be blended). These also give my drink the chilled quality I prefer.

Add green super food supplements to drinks. *(Any brand is fine. Go to your local health food store and search for a brand that you feel good about.) This will turn your drink green or brown depending on ingredients, but it will not affect the flavor.*

Add vegetable protein powder to your drink if you are not eating a protein for breakfast. Or, add nuts as a source of protein. You can add whey or soy protein if your diet allows, but I prefer and suggest the vegetable sources.

Add your favorite green leaf vegetable to drinks. I prefer baby spinach, so I keep a container or bag of fresh spinach in my refrigerator. Kale or Swiss chard is another good option. This will turn your drink green, but will not affect the good flavor. I even add spinach or greens to my fruit drinks.

If you grow fresh herbs, add these for enhanced flavor and nutrition. Some good herbs to use are fresh parsley, basil and cilantro. Fresh ginger is good, too, just use it sparingly.

Samples of My Favorites:

(Note: Use ground flax seeds or chia seeds interchangeably. Flax seeds have a distinct nutty flavor. This will alter the flavor of your drink. Chia seeds do not alter flavor, but they absorb any liquids and expand making your drink thicker. Chia seeds do not need to be ground.)

1. Pineapple, spinach, watercress, parsley, ground flax seed, coconut, almond or rice milk and grapes
2. Watermelon, grape, kiwi, basil, ice and water
3. Banana, peanut/almond butter, rice, almond or coconut milk, chocolate cocoa powder, ground flax seeds
4. Pineapple, mango, orange, spinach, coconut, almond or rice milk and grapes
5. Berries, coconut, almond or rice milk, flax seeds, ice
6. Orange, pineapple, cucumber, carrot and grapes and coconut, almond or rice milk
7. Strawberries, banana, orange and coconut, almond or rice milk, ice
8. Pear, spinach, cucumber, kiwi, grapes, water and ice
9. Tomato, spinach, carrot, celery, cucumber, zucchini, water, ice, parsley and basil

Good foods to use: Pineapple, grapes, banana, mango, berries, cucumber, spinach, kale, pears, beets, skinned lemon or lime, Swiss chard, arugula, watercress, celery, carrots, zucchini or yellow squash, tomato, papaya, kiwi, melons, orange, tangerine, apple, nuts, and coconut.

Sherbet Punch

When you are undergoing chemotherapy, the first priority is comfort and survival. Your body will need optimal calories and nutrients to survive. Sometimes food can't go down, or only with a struggle. Sometimes you need something to just feel good and comforting.

My comfort food and a guaranteed drink that I could handle and made me feel good was sherbet punch.

I would take a large glass and add a scoop of my favorite sherbet. Then fill the glass half-full with organic cranberry juice. Fill the remaining glass with sparkling water and let it sit for a couple of minutes. Add ice and drink through a straw.

Tip: You can eliminate the sherbet and just drink cranberry juice and seltzer water with ice for a very refreshing and hydrating drink. Add clean lemon or lime if you choose for a boost. This is a great drink in a restaurant; (just avoid the lemon or lime due to the possible bacteria present in the commercial preparation of citrus fruits or bring your own).

Tip: Avoid sodas, especially diet sodas and artificial sweeteners. Carry a supply of Stevia sweetener packets or drops in your 'daily travel kit'.

Lemons

Here is a tip and treasure I will bet you probably did not know. Lemons are a little nugget of gold I discovered and they are counter intuitive to common sense. We tend to think of lemons as being acidic, but when they are consumed, they are actually very alkalizing to the body. So, when you consume lemons, they help your digestion, heal heartburn, nausea and indigestion and improve your mood and energy in the process. Lemons are said to help detoxify your body as well.

Just squeeze a half of a well cleaned lemon in water, add the lemon itself and heat to warm.

I recommend warm lemon water in the mornings before eating, or at night before bed to aid your digestive system, immune system and mood. You can also add a small slice of ginger or a splash of Aloe Vera juice. Some people like to add cucumber, too, but I caution that cucumbers in water become very strong very quickly and can upset the stomach.

Snacks

Keep snacks readily available to keep your strength and improve your mood. Nuts or seeds are a good snack since they provide good healthy protein and fats. Chocolate will also help uplift your mood. You can buy high quality granola and nut bars to keep in your car or purse, too.

Tip: I kept granola bars and bags of nuts and seeds in my 'Travel Survival Kit' so I always had a snack available when I got hungry.

Tip: Studies show that dark chocolate is healthy and uplifting. While I use M&M's in this recipe, dark chocolate is a better substitute.

I made my own trail mix to eat and keep with me. You can add or change to your preference. This can also be made in large quantities and stored in the freezer. Or, you can visit Wegman's® grocery store and visit their trail mix bar to make your own. Mix together and transfer to individual bags.

Trail Mix

1 can of your favorite nuts (or mixed nuts)
1 can or jar of sunflower seeds
1 bag of M&Ms or your favorite dark chocolate pieces
1 small jar or bag of raisins or dried cranberries (or both)

Sore Mouth

Please contact your physician if you develop a sore in your mouth. These can be very painful and can lead to infection, so alert your physician immediately.

Foods that are easy on your mouth would be smoothies, baby food, cottage cheese or yogurt, soft boiled or scrambled eggs, banana, applesauce, mashed potatoes or baked sweet potatoes, and pureed soup. (*See my recipes for suggestions.*)

Also, you can suck on ice chips or popsicles to soothe your mouth.

Travel and Daily Management

Travel Survival Kit

I kept a plastic bag of my key survival ingredients in my purse so that I had them with me at all times. For men, consider a small nylon or leather bag to keep in your car, office, or to carry with you. Include:

Peppermint Altoids®

Alcohol swabs

Any prescribed nausea medications

Antibacterial gel and antibacterial wipes

Prescription medications

A thermometer (*Note: It is critical to report a fever as soon as it starts, so I was encouraged to keep a thermometer with me at all times*)

Asthma inhaler (if you have asthma)

Pain patches if prescribed

TUMS® for heartburn or indigestion

Pain relievers

Stevia sweetener packets or drops

Snacks: Trail mix, granola bars, dried fruit, nuts or seeds

High Calorie Supplements

If you have lost weight, or are losing weight in the process, there are enhancements you can use to help you gain caloric content in addition to your diet.

Boost®: You can buy Boost® or Boost Plus® (or equivalent brand) in your local grocery store or pharmacy. Boost® also makes an enhanced drink called *Boost VHC® (Very High Calorie)*. This can be hard to find. This is their very high calorie drink with 530 calories per serving. I found this on www.amazon.com. You can also add this to your smoothies or soups.

ScandiShake®: This is another high calorie alternative. This tastes more like a shake than the others. I also found this on www.amazon.com.

BeneCalorie®: This is a high calorie paste that you can add to food such as soup, smoothies, mashed potatoes, yogurt, cottage cheese or peanut butter. There is little taste, so it does not change the taste of the food you are eating. I also found this on www.Amazon.com.

Quinoa: Quinoa is a grain that has a high caloric content and fiber and is good for you. Use it instead of rice, pasta or potatoes. Cook it with seasonings and vegetable/chicken broth. This is also light and easy on your stomach and digestion.

Nut butters: Put nut butters on anything and everything. Or, just eat it by the spoonful! They are high in protein and will provide the satiety and energy you need.

Pain Medication

If you are prescribed pain medication, especially narcotics, there is a good chance you will experience constipation. If so, get a stool softener from your local pharmacy. Eat high fiber foods and drink lots of fluids. Try to avoid laxatives. Laxatives are harsh and could have damaging side effects.

Tip: Don't forget about the old proven therapy: drink prune juice. This is a safe, natural and guaranteed way to stay regular. I also used magnesium spray or a magnesium liquid like Natural Calm® to ensure regularity. Magnesium is also a great stress reducer and sleep aid, and great for your heart, too. You can find these products at your health food store, Whole Foods® or Wegman's®.

Pain medications may make you sleepy or foggy. These symptoms may reduce over time if you are indeed still in pain. Narcotics seem to be effective when there is real pain, but they can become highly addictive. Please stop taking narcotics when pain subsides or over the counter medications will work.

If you are prescribed a pain medication or appetite enhancement drug that has a mind altering affect (Marinol®), please call for others to drive you where you need to go, or take your medications at night when you are home and safe. Do not drive if you are under the influence of medications.

Grocery Delivery

Please rely on your family and friends to shop for you. This will help you, but will also help them. Most of your friends and family WANT to help, but don't know how. Here is a perfect way for you to tell them "this is how you can help me." They have to shop anyway, so they can pick up your things, too.

If that doesn't work, or you don't have a support system, most major grocery chains have home delivery. I have used Giant's Peapod® service many times. It was especially ideal because they would bring the food (especially heavy items I couldn't carry) up my steps and would put the items in my kitchen. It is totally shop on line so you can make as many changes as you want until midnight before delivery. This was a lifesaver for me for months!

You can go to www.peapod.com to begin your ordering and delivery.

Port

Once you have made the decision to receive chemotherapy, you will have to undergo numerous treatments via IV. There are also numerous blood tests, and depending on your type of cancer, other treatments, biopsies or procedures, too. When I started chemotherapy, I had lymphoma, so I also had numerous blood tests. During the first two rounds of chemotherapy, I found that the veins in my arms were getting dark and taking a long time to heal, plus the pure discomfort of constant sticks were just becoming unbearable.

I chose to have a port inserted in my chest so that all medications could be dispensed through the port, and all blood tests could be rendered from there as well. I recommend you talk to your doctor first.

For me, the port was the best solution, but it may not be for everyone.

Positives

All medications are injected through the port painlessly.

All blood draws are done through the port painlessly.

Some nurses say they appreciate the port because it makes administering the IV much easier for them.

Insurance covers the procedure.

You won't have vein damage in your arms from IV treatments.

There are no issues with finding adequate veins or numerous pricks.

Negatives

This is an outpatient surgical procedure to put it in and take it out.

You have to undergo anesthesia and plan for a 4-6 hour event each time plus a day to recuperate from the anesthesia.

There is pain and soreness for a couple of days after each procedure.

You may need to limit where your procedures happen because the general phlebotomist or nurse cannot withdraw blood through a port. Blood needs to be drawn through an infusion center specialist.

You will have a scar on your chest.

If the port is inserted and placed well, you will have a hard plastic mound implanted underneath your skin that may appear through clothing. This is in the center of one side of your chest midway on your upper rib cage.

The port has to be flushed every 4-6 weeks with heparin, so if you are not in active treatment you will need to go in regularly to have the port flushed with heparin to keep it from clotting and closing off.

You will also need to have the port surgically removed once you have completed your treatment. You will have 2 outpatient procedures in total.

Tip: I recommend that you find a competent surgeon you trust, especially a thoracic surgeon who is experienced in placing these ports. Talk to your oncologist for a surgeon recommendation. If the port is not placed correctly, you may have many unfortunate complications. Fortunately, I had a fabulous surgeon and my port was thoroughly a positive addition to my treatment.

Neulasta®

Your treatment protocol may include a Neulasta® injection to boost your immune system by forcing your body to create new blood cells through the bone marrow. This is a very helpful and positive treatment. However, it is very likely that you may experience intense bone and muscle pain. I found that I would wake up the next day feeling like I got run over by a bus– or I had the flu. Every muscle and bone ached and hurt. This drug is designed to stimulate your bone marrow to produce new blood cells to increase your immunity. Neulasta® is part of some chemotherapy treatments where it is important to protect you from infection if your immune system becomes compromised from chemotherapy.

I don't know why, but I was told to take 4 Advil® every 4-8 hours and 1 Claritin® every day. I was told not to change brands. Again, I don't know why, but I followed the instructions, and it did help.

Tip: Take the Claritin® and Advil® beginning the night before your treatment. Also, I found that sitting and lying down only enhanced the discomfort. I used this time to walk around and move as much as possible to diminish the muscle aches.

Sleep/Naps

The best thing you can do is surrender to the process. You should expect that you will be tired with low energy. You should be loving and kind to yourself and know there is an end point, but in the process, just rest. Don't force your body to do more than it can because it's working overtime to heal you. Just make your bed a safe and very comfortable place. Live there if you need to, like I did. Sleep as often as you need, no matter what the hour. I found I was like a mother with a newborn child. I would wake and sleep on 3-4 hour intervals. I didn't fight it. I gave into it and slept when I needed, and used my waking hours to eat, stay connected to my friends and family, and found contentment in games and books on my Kindle or laptop. I also recorded my favorite TV shows on my DVR so that I could watch them during my waking hours. Often, this would be in the middle of the night.

Tip: Melatonin is a natural remedy to help you sleep. It is non-addictive and will not give you a hangover or mind fog. You can buy this at any pharmacy. I also used Calmes Forte® natural sleeping remedy. It does really help to get a good night's sleep. Sleep is SO essential to healing. Please speak with your doctor about any sleep supplements or medications to make sure they are not interacting with any other medications you might be taking.

Germ Prevention

If you are undergoing chemotherapy, then your immune system will more than likely be compromised. Please talk to your oncologist in detail about the level of protection you need.

I kept a medicine cabinet in my purse in a plastic bag. It contained a small package of disinfectant wipes and antibacterial gel that I used every time I went anywhere. (*See my Travel Survival Kit*).

Keep in mind seemingly common or friendly places:

Telephones: no matter where you go, pull out a wipe and wash it down.

Door knobs: yes, wipe them (and your hands) down as you leave.

Computer keyboards, cell phones, steering wheels, remote controls, and faucets.

ATM machines, gas dispensing nozzles, elevators and grocery carts.

Air Travel: unless your doctor advises, you don't need a facemask, but I highly recommend that when you board the plane and take your seat, pull out a wipe, add antibacterial gel to it and wipe down your armrests, tray tables and everything solid in your seating area.

If you are eating in a restaurant, take a wipe and wipe down your table, the salt and pepper shakers, condiments and menu.

Do not order lemons or limes in a restaurant. They are a breeding ground of bacteria. They are sliced and sit together in a container. You can't be sure if they've been washed, and how many hands have been in the container. I would just avoid them altogether or bring your own.

Do not get a professional manicure or pedicure during chemotherapy since you could develop an infection if scraped or cut.

Avoid raw fish; i.e. sushi, due to possible mercury levels or possible infection.

Avoid any dental procedures during chemotherapy, since there is a potential to develop an infection if any tissue becomes exposed. Also, use a soft gentle toothbrush to avoid any irritation to gums or mouth tissue. Use a gentle alcohol free mouthwash.

Tip: Schedule a dental cleaning and manicure/pedicure prior to entering chemotherapy if you are able.

Alternative Therapies

If you have the opportunity to take advantage of therapeutic massages or energy healing services, I would highly recommend you utilize any or all that interest you. Your goal is to heal physically, emotionally and spiritually. Suggestions may include therapeutic massage, energy healing, Healing Touch, Reiki, gentle Yoga, and meditation.

I especially liked Trager® massage because it is so gentle and restores your body's natural movements and processes. I began this just a couple of weeks after my major thoracic surgery and still continue today. I contribute a large part of my healing to this process.

I also really enjoyed any form of energy healing therapy including Healing Touch, Bethesda Natural Healing Therapy® and Reiki.

Check your local hospital or community cancer support facilities to see what options may be available for you. You can also check your local community listings for providers in your area.

You can also go to www.mindpower3.com for many excellent guided meditation or brain entrainment programs.

Attitude

I cannot emphasize enough the importance and power of a positive attitude. During the entire process, I sent loving and healing thoughts to my body, my providers and caregivers and *expected* healing as an outcome. I spent my days giving gratitude and thanks for everything I could find. This process softened me and made me more open to all of the possibilities of healing. While my circumstances were dire when I was going through the process, I focused on "thanking God for a true healing experience." I did not think about or focus on the misery I was experiencing. And, it worked, because I am here today, healthy and happy to share my hope and my life with you.

Prayer and Meditation

I am not advocating any religious or spiritual bias. I do feel that a close connection with a Higher Power or the God of your understanding is very important throughout the healing process.

Meditation will help calm fear, induce a state of relaxation and can enhance any experience. If you are not familiar with meditation, you can go to www.mindpower3.com and use any of the music or guided meditations to assist you.

Tip: There are free samples you can use to download onto your laptop or mobile device to use during your treatments, or when you are home and need to reduce stress or relax to a sleep state.

TV/iPad/Kindle/Smart Phone

In our current age of technology, I found having a smart phone and portable device like a Kindle® or iPad® imperative. Many waiting rooms carry limited magazines or newspapers now. And, many hours are spent in doctors' offices or infusion centers. I always brought a small bag with my devices or any books or magazines I wanted to read.

If there is a particular magazine you like, subscribe to it either in paper form or on your Kindle® or Nook®. Download books you want to read so you always have something to read while you are waiting–you will do a LOT of waiting!

Tip: If you are a loved one, buy a subscription to their favorite magazine.

Tip: If you are a loved one, and have the financial means, buy them a media reader device like a Kindle Fire® or Nook®.

Social Contact

Isolation is a real challenge for anyone that is ill. Social contact is so critical to health and emotional well-being. Undergoing cancer therapy and feeling tired or sick can be very isolating and depressing. Allow yourself to do whatever is necessary to feel better. Listen to your body and allow yourself to heal without forcing yourself to do more than you can handle. This is easier said than done, sometimes. Stay in contact with close supporters and loved ones, even if it's only on the phone, when you have the energy. There are also chat rooms and support rooms on the internet if you are not mobile.

Also, I highly recommend a support group in your community where you can connect with people that share your situation. Every community has them. Ask your doctor or infusion center.

Tip: Talk to your nurses, doctors, technicians and caregivers. Engage them. They love to care for you and share in your life. Share in theirs, too. Get to know them. This will help you feel connected.

Exercise

If you are able to walk, or do gentle Yoga stretching, this will help keep your energy elevated and enhance healing. This will also help the quality of your sleep.

If you have been engaged in physical therapy from your surgery or treatments, keep it up, and do your 'homework' to keep your strength and energy going.

I found that the best thing for me was to go outside and walk. Often this was only 5-10 minutes, but just breathing in fresh air, moving my body, and getting away from the 'walls that I was confined to' really helped my physical and emotional strength.

Diary/eMail Updates/Journaling

Keep a daily diary of your events, either through writing in a journal or sending email updates. This will help you to channel your experience and emotions. You will also have this to look back on once you have finished. This is a very healing energy practice.

Write letters to your loved ones. This is such a healing practice. You will give them a legacy, and they will feel your love and appreciation. Their love and appreciation will come back to strengthen you.

Gratitude

I know the last thing you want to hear is me telling you to be grateful for cancer and chemotherapy.

Please trust me. The single BEST thing you can do is surrender and say thank you at all times to your body for surviving the chemotherapy and treatments, and for giving you the experience of true healing. Your body will survive because that is what it's meant to do. Also, constantly thank your physicians, nurses, family members, friends, care givers and technicians. They will appreciate it, and they will give back so much more.

Cancer may bring the best of times and the worst of times.

You may become close to some, and lose support from others you thought were close. This is common. Some people will fall away because of fear. Let them go with love and acceptance. God, or your Higher Power, will bring others; new people to help you through this journey. Don't harbor resentment.

Trust that you will always have the right people you need through this process.

How Family and Friends Can Help

Many people ask and wonder how they can help a friend or loved one with cancer. Everyone's situation will be different, but I've listed some excellent suggestions and ideas.

Order a Maid Service: I lived alone and did not have live-in family to do my chores. A good friend of mine ordered a maid service to come and clean my home. This was marvelous since I did not have the strength or energy to clean, or run a vacuum, or scrub bathtubs. You can find high quality cleaning services on the internet. Many will do one time cleanings or multiple cleanings. If you can't afford to order a maid service, offer to provide some of the cleaning yourself.

Volunteer to Drive: Some procedures will require that the patient be driven and picked up from a procedure due to anesthesia. This is a critical need for many patients.

Volunteer to Shop: If you need to go to the grocery store (and I know you do) offer to pick up items for your friend and take them to their home.

Take them for a Haircut: Most cancer patients cannot have manicures or pedicures due to infection control, but they will need and want a haircut. Schedule this for them, and take them. This will be a great way for you to bond, share time together, and help break their isolation.

Volunteer to Babysit or Take Kids: As I mentioned earlier, energy levels will probably be very low. Children, and their obligations, can be a drain and responsibility too great to handle at times. Sleep is important. Volunteer to take children to allow for a much needed nap.

Visit: As I have mentioned before, isolation and loneliness are VERY real for people undergoing treatment. Bring your presence and company. There is nothing more uplifting to a patient than a smile and conversation with others. Get them out of the home if you can, even if it's to a park or coffee shop.

Volunteer to Run Errands: Life doesn't stop when cancer strikes. There are so many little things and loose ends that need to happen. Maybe it's going to the post office, or taking the clothes to the dry cleaner. The ideas are endless. If you are going to be running errands for yourself, call and see if any of these would be helpful for your friend or family member.

Meet for Lunch or Coffee: There is nothing more pleasing to a patient than company, getting out of the house and having a sense of engaging in life. Meet for an hour to let them know you care.

Notes/Cards/emails: If you do not live nearby, send occasional cards, letters or emails. These are so uplifting and provide a sense of belonging. If you feel pressed for time, or are unsure of what to say, just send a one line email: "Hi, I just wanted to let you know I was thinking about you. Hang in there. Love, me."

Bring or Help Prepare Food: Anything you can do to help your friend or family member get through treatment is welcomed. Food is big for people in treatment. The only suggestion I would make is *ask what they would like, and what they can eat*. Do not assume, or bring YOUR favorite food. They may have diet restrictions, food aversions or cravings. They may have nausea limiting the kind of food they can handle. Don't assume chicken noodle soup.

Take them for a Massage or Energy Healing Session: Some communities, like mine, have not-for-profit organizations that provide amazing services for cancer patients. Take them for healing and therapy sessions.

Drive to Support Groups: Offer to drive them to a cancer support group.

Pick Up Their Laundry: Anything you can do to minimize strenuous chores is so incredible. Do their laundry, ironing or dry cleaning. Bring it back folded and clean. Amazing!

Handy Man or Woman: If you are handy around the house, or are competent at 'fixing things', offer your time. Change light bulbs, batteries, clean air filters, sweep the garage or porch or cut the grass.

Walk the Dog or Play with Kids: Send your pre-teen or teenager to play with young children and/or walk the dog.

Local Support Groups

Ask your oncologist or infusion center about local cancer support groups. They are so helpful on so many levels. Mainly, they will help you break the feeling of isolation and help you feel connected to others that are experiencing the same conditions.

I can't recommend this enough. If you need transportation, call your local support group and ask for a ride, or spend the money to get a taxi cab. Someone from your group will surely love to drive you home.

Tip: This is an excellent way for family and friends to offer help.

I am blessed with the opportunity to be living in a community with a non-profit organization that provides services to cancer patients free of charge. I use and support *The Wellness House of Annapolis.* They provide support groups, healing therapies, nutritional programs and counseling services for cancer patients. Check to see if your local community has a similar support organization.

Professional Counseling Support

There are licensed counselors who specialize in dealing with cancer patients. I would highly encourage you to find a therapist that specializes in cancer. They can help combat depression, isolation, anger, and other issues that are central to cancer patients. If you are terminal, they are also excellent at helping you plan your last days.

Please ask your oncologist for a referral. If they do not know, then contact your local not-for-profit support agency. At last resort, go to the internet and search for a therapist who specializes in cancer therapy.

Live Fearlessly With Cancer©

I have created a cancer support website on www.livefearlesslywithcancer.com and a group Facebook® page where you can chat with others, gain other support services and resources or buy this book and future books. Go to my website for all links to services.

Please help me to spread the word. My mission is to make resources and support services available to every single person dealing with cancer or chronic illness.

Please support my mission by spreading the word.

Other Support Organizations and Resources

National Cancer Institute

1-800-4-CANCER (800-422-6237)

www.cancer.gov

Chat www.cancer.gov/livehelp

American Cancer Society

1-800-ACS-2345 (800-227-2345)

www.cancer.org

Cancer Support Community

1-888-793-9355

www.cancersupportcommunity.org

CancerCare, Inc.

1-800-813-HOPE (1-800-813-4673)

www.cancercare.org

National Institute of Health

www.nih.gov

Health Information: www.health.nih.gov

Epilogue

I would like to thank all of my family, friends, caregivers, doctors, nurses, technicians and therapists for their time, talents, love and care. I could not have made it through without you. I thank God for all of you every day.

I hope that you found something in this book to help ease your burden. If you are a family member or friend, I hope you found a way to help and learned something about the cancer treatment experience.

I'm in the process of building a website to offer free additional information and services to anyone with cancer, or anyone who wants to support someone with cancer or chronic illness. I will be continually offering other products and services to help cancer patients and their family members thrive and survive. Stay tuned! I'm always transforming, and building.

Live fearlessly!

Jennifer

Dedication

I dedicate this book, and this labor of my love, to repay and honor my mother. She is my soul mate, best friend and supporter. She gave to me all she had when there was nothing left. She has been unconditional in her love for me. She is my diamond.